HERBS FOR EXCESSIVE SWEATING

Nature's Soothing Solutions, Unlocking The Power To Conquer Hotness Naturally Through Cooling Herbal Remedies

DR. JEREMY ALLEY

Copyright © DR. JEREMY ALLEY 2024

All rights reserved. No part of this publication may be reproduced, distributed, or transmitted in any form or by any means, including photocopying, recording, or other electronic or mechanical methods, without the prior written permission of the author, except in the case of brief quotations embodied in critical reviews and certain other noncommercial uses permitted by copyright law.

Disclaimer:

The information provided in this book, is intended for general informational purposes only and should not be considered as professional advice.

The author has made every effort to ensure the accuracy of the information presented. However, readers are advised to consult with a qualified healthcare professional before attempting any herbal remedies or making significant changes to their wellness routine. Individual health conditions vary, and what may be suitable for one person may not be appropriate for another.

It is important to note that the author is not in any endorsement deal, partnership, or affiliation with any organization, brand, or company mentioned in this book. Any references to specific products or services are based on the author's personal experience or general knowledge and do not imply an endorsement or promotion of those products or services.

Contents

Overview

Hyperhidrosis, the medical term for excessive sweating, is a disorder that affects a considerable number of people globally. Sweating excessively and uncontrollably can cause discomfort, embarrassment, and in rare cases, social anxiety. Even though there are many traditional therapies for excessive perspiration, more and more people are using herbal remedies as a cure. This book explores the potential advantages of using herbal treatments to manage and reduce excessive perspiration.

About This Book

Welcome to a thorough instruction on using herbs to treat excessive perspiration. The goal of this book is to give readers insightful information on natural remedies that could help them deal with the problems associated with excessive and chronic sweating. We welcome you to embark on a journey to find alternate approaches to managing this ailment and enhancing your general well-being as we delve into the world of herbal treatments.

Comprehending Abnormal Sweating

It is essential to comprehend excessive sweating and its underlying causes to treat the illness properly. This section explores the different causes of hyperhidrosis, which include hormonal imbalances, heredity, and medical problems. People can investigate the potential advantages of herbal remedies and make well-informed judgments about their treatment options by developing a greater awareness of excessive perspiration.

Meaning and Reasons

Sweating excessively goes beyond the body's typical reaction to heat or physical activity. A thorough definition of hyperhidrosis is given in this section, with a distinction made between the primary and secondary types of the disorder. Moreover, it delves into the various reasons behind excessive perspiration, illuminating how elements like stress, food, and underlying medical conditions can exacerbate this difficult and sometimes misdiagnosed ailment.

The Value of Herbal Remedies

Herbal medicines are becoming more and more popular, therefore it's important to understand how important they are for treating excessive perspiration. This section examines the benefits of using herbal remedies, highlighting their all-natural and comprehensive approach to symptom management. For those looking for alternatives to traditional treatments, herbal therapies present a viable path due to their potential to reduce sweating and improve general skin health.

We shall explore particular herbs that are effective in treating excessive perspiration in the upcoming chapters. Every plant will be thoroughly examined, covering its background, possible modes of action, and useful applications. By the time this book ends, readers will have learned a lot about how to use herbal remedies in their daily lives to live a more comfortable and balanced life even in the face of problems caused by excessive perspiration.

CHAPTER ONE

THE ESSENTIALS OF OVERDUE SWEATING

Hyperhidrosis, often known as excessive sweating, is a medical disorder marked by sweat production that exceeds what is required for adequate thermoregulation.

Although sweating is a normal and necessary biological process that helps the body cool down, those who have hyperhidrosis have excessive sweating.

This can happen in the hands, feet, face, and underarms, among other places on the body.

There are several potential causes for hyperhidrosis, including underlying medical disorders and hereditary factors.

Synopsis Of Hyperhidrosis

A deeper examination of hyperhidrosis's prevalence, causes, and possible triggers is necessary to comprehend the condition. People of all ages and genders may be impacted by this illness, which can hurt their quality of life generally, social relationships, and emotional health. Certain medical illnesses, including diabetes, thyroid problems, or nervous system disorders, may be connected to certain types of hyperhidrosis. Addressing both the physical and psychological elements of hyperhidrosis is crucial since emotional stress and worry can worsen symptoms.

Various Forms Of Abnormal Sweating

There are various ways that hyperhidrosis might present itself, but primary focal hyperhidrosis is the most typical.

This kind of profuse perspiration is restricted to particular regions, including the cheeks, underarms, palms, and soles of the feet.

Conversely, secondary global hyperhidrosis is linked to an underlying illness or medicine. Investigating these differences is essential to creating focused and potent herbal remedies suited to each person's unique hyperhidrosis type and severity.

Effects On Day-To-Day Living

Hyperhidrosis has effects that go beyond discomfort. People who have this illness frequently experience difficulties in their daily lives, both in social and professional contexts.

Sweating all the time might cause self-consciousness, social scenario avoidance, and low self-esteem.

The need to hide sweat stains may have an impact on the selection of clothes, thus reducing the amount of clothing possibilities.

'Occupational difficulties can occur, particularly in positions requiring a lot of face-to-face communication. It is essential to address how hyperhidrosis affects day-to-day functioning while creating holistic herbal remedies that support mental and physical health.

CHAPTER TWO

AN EXPLORATION OF HERBAL REMEDIES

Hyperhidrosis, or excessive sweating, is a common ailment that can make sufferers feel uncomfortable and ashamed. Herbal therapies provide a natural and comprehensive way to treat excessive sweating, even though there are many conventional treatments available. For those looking for alternatives to conventional procedures, it is essential to comprehend the underlying theories of herbal remedies.

Herbal Medicine's Power

For millennia, herbal medicine has been an integral part of traditional healing methods in many countries. Herbs are powerful because they contain a wide range of bioactive chemicals that can be used therapeutically.

Certain herbs are recognized for their astringent and cooling qualities, which can assist in controlling the body's natural cooling system when excessive perspiration occurs without interfering with physiological functions.

The Operation Of Herbal Remedies

The primary way that herbal treatments for excessive sweating work is because of their distinct biochemical makeup.

Many herbs have inherent astringent qualities that can aid in constricting sweat glands to lessen perspiration production. Herbs having adaptogenic qualities may also aid in controlling the body's reaction to stress, which is frequently the cause of excessive perspiration.

Comprehending the mechanisms of action underlying herbal remedies offers valuable insight into their efficacy, enabling folks to make well-informed decisions regarding their use.

Benefits Of Herbal Remedies

Choosing herbal therapies to treat excessive perspiration has several benefits. Herbal remedies tend to be kinder to the body than some conventional medicines, which might have unfavorable side effects.

They are good for people with delicate skin or those who are allergic to things because they usually cause fewer negative effects.

Furthermore, because herbal medicine is holistic, it treats underlying imbalances that lead to excessive sweating in addition to the symptoms.

This all-encompassing strategy may result in long-term alleviation and enhanced general well-being.

Investigating herbal therapies for excessive perspiration entails learning about the medicinal properties of herbs, their physiological action, and their unique benefits. Herbal remedies show up as a viable, all-encompassing choice that works with the body's natural cycles as more people look for alternate methods of controlling their excessive perspiration.

CHAPTER THREE

DETERMINING RISK AND CHANGES IN LIFESTYLE

Effective management of excessive sweating requires knowledge of the triggers. To find relief, it can be important to understand the triggers that lead to increased perspiration, which will be covered in detail in this section. Modifying one's lifestyle is crucial, and this part will assist readers in forming routines that can reduce excessive perspiration.

Typical Causes Of Excessive Sweating

Excessive sweating can be caused by a variety of things, from underlying medical disorders to environmental variables. This section of the manual will go into more detail about these triggers, illuminating the physiological and environmental elements that might make hyperhidrosis worse. It is necessary to identify these triggers to apply focused herbal therapies.

Changes In Lifestyle To Control Sweating

We'll look at several lifestyle changes in this part that can help control excessive perspiration. Readers will find helpful advice for incorporating these adjustments into their everyday activities, from dressing appropriately to using stress-reduction tactics. Changing one's lifestyle is frequently the first step towards treating the underlying reasons for excessive perspiration.

Dietary Suggestions

Overall health is greatly influenced by diet, and particular foods can either cause or lessen excessive perspiration.

In this episode, we'll discuss dietary suggestions that try to harmonize the body's internal functions to lower the risk of hyperhidrosis. We'll also talk about herbal medicines and teas that work well with dietary modifications to treat excessive perspiration holistically.

With so many people looking for natural ways to deal with excessive sweating, this article attempts to give a thorough understanding of the available herbal remedies.

By adopting these solutions into their daily routine, people can alleviate the difficulties caused by hyperhidrosis and enhance their general well-being.

CHAPTER FOUR

HERBS FOR THE INTERNAL SYSTEM

Restoring equilibrium within is crucial to controlling excessive perspiration. Herbs are known to be adaptogenic, such as ashwagandha and Rhodiola, and aid in controlling how the body reacts to stress, which is frequently the cause of increased sweating. By supporting hormonal balance, these herbs lessen the chance of hyperactive sweat glands.

Moreover, sage has been used traditionally to reduce perspiration due to its astringent qualities. Its organic ingredients have antiperspirant properties that reduce excessive sweating. Including these herbs in your regular regimen can help create a more harmonious atmosphere within.

Herbal Infusions And Teas

Herbal teas offer a calming and practical solution for controlling excessive perspiration. Particularly noteworthy for its capacity to lessen perspiration production is sage tea. Making a pot of sage tea and drinking it daily can be an easy but useful addition to your regimen.

Furthermore, peppermint tea has cooling properties that might assist in controlling body temperature and possibly lessen the need to perspire excessively. Adding these herbal infusions to your regular water intake offers a delicious and all-natural way to combat hyperhidrosis.

Supplements And Tinctures

Supplements and herbal tinctures can be powerful partners in the fight against excessive perspiration. With its astringent qualities, witch hazel can be consumed internally or applied topically to help regulate sweat production and tighten pores.

Additionally, taking burdock root supplements aids the body's detoxification processes by removing toxins that could be causing excessive perspiration. Including these herbal remedies in your wellness routine will offer all-encompassing assistance in controlling hyperhidrosis.

Including Herbs In Your Nutrition

Herbs are a great way to control your excessive perspiration without going overboard. Because of its high chlorophyll content, cilantro works as a natural deodorant to eliminate body smells brought on by perspiration. Fresh cilantro may be a tasty and nutritious addition to smoothies or salads.

Additionally, adding turmeric to your food not only boosts flavor but also benefits from its anti-inflammatory qualities, which may help minimize perspiration.

These culinary herbs improve the flavor and nutritious content of your meals while offering a pleasurable solution to excessive sweating.

Herbal remedies for excessive perspiration provide a healthy, all-natural substitute for pharmaceutical therapies.

You can take a thorough approach to controlling hyperhidrosis and enhancing general well-being by taking care of internal balance, embracing herbal teas, investigating tinctures and supplements, and including herbs in your diet.

Topical Herbal Remedies

For many people, excessive sweating, or hyperhidrosis, can be a chronic and uncomfortable condition. Applying topical herbal remedies is one way to address this problem. Many herbs have inherent antiperspirant and astringent qualities that might help reduce perspiration.

For example, sage has chemicals that might shrink sweat glands and lessen excessive sweating. Sage leaves can be infused with hot water to make a topical remedy. After the mixture cools, it can be applied topically to the affected areas.

Powdered And Pasted Herbs

Herbal pastes and powders provide an additional efficient way to treat excessive perspiration.

You may make a natural powder that absorbs moisture and neutralizes odor by mixing ingredients like baking soda, arrowroot powder, and crushed herbs like lavender or chamomile.

This powdered herb leaves regions that sweat easily feeling dry and renewed.

Herbal pastes, which are created by combining finely crushed herbs with aloe vera gel or water, can also be applied topically to the skin to provide a cooling and sweat-controlling effect.

Homemade Herbal Sprays For Sweat Relief

Easy to make at home, DIY herbal sweat-reducing sprays provide a quick and refreshing fix. Herbal elements such as peppermint, witch hazel, and aloe vera can be combined to create a cooling and perspiration-controlling spray. These plants have astringent qualities that assist in closing pores and decrease perspiration. Herbal sprays are a useful and transportable solution for usage on the go that is made by blending herbal extracts or essential oils with a base like witch hazel or distilled water.

Herbal Baths To Reduce Perspiration

Including herbal baths in a regular self-care regimen can help relieve general perspiration. Some herbs, like calendula, chamomile, and lavender, have calming qualities that can help regulate the body's sweating process.

One can infuse these herbs into warm bathwater and soak them for approximately 20 minutes to reap the benefits of herbal baths. In addition to reducing excessive perspiration, the herbs' soothing and astringent properties can offer a restful and revitalizing experience.

It's important to be careful of personal sensitivities and allergies, just like with any herbal medicine. It is advisable to speak with a healthcare provider or herbalist before using any new herbal remedies for excessive sweating, particularly if you have any pre-existing problems or are worried about possible interactions.

Including these herbal remedies in a holistic lifestyle that also includes good nutrition and hygiene practices can help manage excessive perspiration naturally.

CHAPTER FIVE

AROMATHERAPY FOR OVERINDULGENT PERSPIRATION

For many people, excessive sweating, or hyperhidrosis, can be an embarrassing and uncomfortable condition. An all-natural solution to controlling excessive sweating is provided by aromatherapy, the therapeutic application of essential oils.

Through the utilization of plant-derived essences, people can effectively tackle the underlying cause of the problem and encourage a state of equilibrium inside their bodies.

Essential Oils For Reducing Sweat

It has been shown that some essential oils have qualities that can assist in regulating excessive perspiration. Because of its antibacterial qualities, tea tree oil can be especially useful in battling the germs that cause sweat-related body odor. Another useful choice is sage oil, which has astringent qualities and helps control the activity of sweat glands. Famous for its relaxing properties, lavender oil not only smells good but also helps reduce tension, which is frequently connected to excessive perspiration.

Methods Of Blending And Application

Making your custom blend of essential oils is an important first step in using aromatherapy for excessive perspiration.

Oils having complementary qualities can be combined to increase their efficacy.

A common combination is a few drops of diluted tea tree, sage, and lavender oils mixed with jojoba or coconut oil.

This blend can offer a pleasant and refreshing remedy when applied to sweat-prone regions like the foot or underarms.

Establishing A Calm Ambience

In addition to direct application, using essential oils to create a calming atmosphere will help reduce general stress, which in turn can help control excessive perspiration.

In living areas, diffusing essential oils such as peppermint, chamomile, or lavender can help create a relaxing mood.

The calming scent may benefit the neurological system by lowering tension and, as a result, the chance of excessive perspiration.

An enjoyable and all-natural solution to the problem of excessive sweating is provided by aromatherapy.

People can control perspiration while taking advantage of aromatherapy's therapeutic effects by adding essential oils with antibacterial and astringent qualities into custom blends and establishing a calming environment.

This all-encompassing method takes into account the psychological health of individuals who experience excessive perspiration in addition to treating the physical symptoms.

CHAPTER SIX

HOLISTIC METHODS

For many people, excessive sweating, or hyperhidrosis, can be embarrassing and uncomfortable.

Even though there are many traditional therapies for this problem, some people go for herbal and alternative remedies. For the management of excessive sweating, holistic approaches—which combine lifestyle modifications and herbal remedies—can provide a more thorough and long-lasting solution.

Breathing Exercises And Yoga

One way to help control excessive sweating is to incorporate breathing exercises and yoga into your routine. Yoga encourages balance and general well-being in the body. Some poses also help to regulate the neurological system, which affects perspiration regulation. Furthermore, targeted breathing techniques like deep diaphragmatic breathing can assist in relaxing the nervous system and lessen the chance of excessive perspiration.

Techniques For Stress Management

Stress and worry are frequently associated with excessive sweating. Sweating bouts may decrease with the use of stress management strategies.

Methods like progressive muscle relaxation, biofeedback, and mindfulness meditation can help people better control their stress levels, which will in turn affect how severe their excessive perspiration is.

These methods offer a comprehensive approach to stress management by treating the underlying cause of the disease.

The Relationship Between The Mind And Body

Sweating is one of the many physiological processes for which the mind-body link is vital. Herbal remedies that focus on the mind-body link may help treat excessive perspiration.

Herbs that are known to help the body adapt to stressors, such as Rhodiola and ashwagandha, are known as adaptogens.

This helps the body reduce the triggers that cause excessive perspiration. These herbs support the body's resilience and equilibrium by acting holistically.

Herbal remedies for excessive perspiration require a comprehensive strategy that takes mental and physical health into account.

Through the integration of techniques such as yoga, breathing exercises, and stress management, people can foster a more harmonic and balanced connection between their mind and body. Herbal treatments that focus on the mind-body connection can also help control excessive perspiration sustainably and naturally.

CHAPTER SEVEN

SUCCESS STORIES AND CASE STUDIES

Analyzing case studies and success stories is one method of evaluating the efficacy of herbal remedies. Real-world examples offer insightful information about how people have included herbal treatments in their daily routines and the results they have achieved. These anecdotes highlight the variety of ways that herbal remedies can improve the quality of life for people who experience excessive perspiration.

Actual Experiences

Studying actual cases is crucial to developing a greater comprehension of the usefulness of employing herbal therapies. This section explores firsthand stories from people who have opted to treat their excessive perspiration using herbal remedies. These stories illustrate the difficulties encountered, the process of making decisions, and the results attained with herbal remedies.

Testimonies From People Who Received Assistance

Testimonials are essential for presenting the subjective experiences of people who have used herbal medicines to relieve their excessive perspiration.

These first-person stories provide an insight into the process of finding and using herbal remedies in day-to-day living. Comprehending the viewpoints of individuals who have profited from these treatments might furnish significant insights for others contemplating analogous methodologies.

For those looking for a natural and organic way to treat their excessive perspiration, herbal remedies offer a viable option.

Together, case studies, firsthand accounts, and testimonies provide a thorough grasp of the beneficial effects herbal medicines have had on the lives of people with hyperhidrosis. Investigating these herbal remedies may present a viable solution to control excessive perspiration in a way that is consistent with a more organic and all-encompassing approach to well-being, even though individual results may differ.

CHAPTER EIGHT

SPEAKING WITH MEDICAL PROFESSIONALS

It is important to speak with medical professionals before attempting to treat excessive sweating. This will help to establish a precise diagnosis and rule out any underlying medical disorders that could be causing the problem. The right course of action is determined by a healthcare professional's thorough assessment, which guarantees the safe and efficient integration of herbal treatments into the entire treatment plan.

Combining Medical Advice With Herbal Remedies

When combined with medical advice, herbal remedies can be a useful supplement to the management of excessive perspiration. Speaking with medical specialists enables a thorough grasp of the patient's condition and guarantees that using herbal medicines won't conflict with any current prescriptions or treatments. By addressing excessive sweating from several perspectives, this integrated method seeks to offer a comprehensive and individualized solution.

Finding Appropriate Herbal Treatments

Herbal remedies have long been used to treat excessive perspiration.

For instance, sage has been utilized to lessen sweat production because of its astringent qualities. Furthermore, witch hazel can be administered topically to regulate perspiration in particular locations due to its inherent anti-inflammatory qualities.

Knowing the particular advantages and uses of any herbal treatment enables people to customize their strategy to meet their own needs.

Modifications To Lifestyle And Herbal Remedies

Changing one's lifestyle can help manage excessive perspiration in general, in addition to integrating natural therapies. Modifying one's lifestyle to avoid triggers like spicy meals and caffeine, wearing loose-fitting clothing, and maintaining proper hygiene can support the herbal approach. To encourage internal equilibrium and lessen excessive sweating, incorporate herbal drinks into your regular regimen, including sage tea.

When To Get Expert Assistance

While many people who suffer from excessive perspiration find success with herbal remedies, it's important to know when seeking professional medical attention is required. Seeking immediate medical assistance is essential if lifestyle changes and herbal medicines are insufficient to relieve the excessive sweating, or if the excessive sweating is accompanied by other worrisome symptoms. When necessary, medical professionals can carry out additional research and suggest cutting-edge therapies or procedures.

When used carefully and after consulting medical professionals, herbal remedies can be an effective way to control excessive perspiration.

Combining these therapies with medical advice gives people a customized, all-encompassing approach to dealing with the problems that come with excessive perspiration. A balance that supports comfort and general well-being can be found by people by combining herbal remedies, lifestyle modifications, and expert advice.

Creating Your Customized Herbal Program

For many people, excessive sweating, or hyperhidrosis, can be an uncomfortable and socially awkward condition. Even though there are many traditional therapies for this problem, some people look for herbal remedies. Choosing herbs that can assist in controlling the body's sweat production and comprehending the underlying causes of excessive perspiration are essential steps in creating a customized herbal regimen.

Establishing A Schedule

When using herbal medicines to control excessive perspiration in your daily life, it's important to establish a regimen.

The secret is to be consistent. You can increase the efficacy of topical applications or herbal consumption by creating a regimen. Incorporating lifestyle modifications like dietary adjustments and stress-reduction tactics into a routine can also help herbal medicines address the underlying causes of excessive perspiration.

Monitoring Development

To ascertain the efficacy of your herbal regimen, you must track and assess its advancement. Note any reduction in symptoms, changes in sweating patterns, and possible side effects in great detail. You can use this tracking technique to help you decide whether to stick to the present herbal plan make changes, or look into alternative medicines. Continually evaluating yourself allows you to remain aware of how your body reacts to herbal remedies.

Modifying Plans Over Time

Understanding that herbal remedies might need to be adjusted over time is essential for long-term success in controlling excessive perspiration. The way the body reacts to herbs might vary, and the potency of the selected herbs can be impacted by variables like stress levels, seasonal variations, and general health. It is important to keep your herbal strategy flexible so that it can be adjusted to your unique demands as they arise.

People can investigate natural solutions to deal with excessive sweating by developing a personalized herbal strategy, setting up a regimen, monitoring progress, and making adjustments over time. It's crucial to speak with medical specialists or herbalists to make sure the herbs you've picked are safe and suitable for your particular circumstance.

FINAL VERDICT

In summary, herbal remedies for excessive perspiration offer a safe, all-natural substitute for traditional therapies. Herbs such as sage, witch hazel, and burdock root can be included in daily routines to address the underlying causes of hyperhidrosis. Individual reactions to herbal medicines can differ, so it's vital to remember that speaking with a healthcare provider is advised, particularly for people who may already have underlying medical issues. Adopting these herbal remedies could provide comfort to people looking for a comprehensive and long-term solution to control their excessive perspiration.

Summary Of Important Ideas

There are several reasons why people sweat excessively or develop hyperhidrosis, including hormonal abnormalities and genetics.

Herbal therapies for the underlying reasons of excessive perspiration include sage, witch hazel, and burdock root.

Sage controls sweat gland activity and functions as a natural antiperspirant.

When applied topically, witch hazel's astringent qualities aid in reducing excessive perspiration and tightening pores.

The cleansing qualities of burdock root improve general health and may lessen perspiration by treating internal imbalances.

Motivation For The Upcoming Trip

It takes perseverance and patience to start using herbal medicines to treat excessive perspiration. Whether as topicals, teas, or supplements, these herbs must be incorporated into everyday life. Although each person will react differently, the all-encompassing quality of herbal remedies provides a mild and long-lasting way to address the problems caused by excessive perspiration. As you progress toward natural well-being, never lose hope.